CARB CYCLING FOR WEIGHT LOSS FOR ENDOMORPH WOMEN

A Guide For Endomorph

Maria D. Johnson

TABLE OF CONTENT

INTRODUCTION...4

CHAPTER 1...7
UNDERSTANDING ENDOMORPHS.................. 7
❖ **What Makes You an Endomorph?**.................7

CHAPTER 2.. 10
THE POWER OF CARB CYCLING................... 10
❖ **How Carb Cycling Helps Endomorph Women.**
10

CHAPTER 3...14
STARTING YOUR CARB CYCLING JOURNEY..14
❖ **Assessing Your Current Diet and Goals**........14

CHAPTER 4.. 18
CRAFTING YOUR CARB CYCLING DIET..........18
❖ **Choosing Carbs Wisely**...............................18

CHAPTER 5.. 23
Meal Plans Made Easy................................. 23
❖ **Sample Meals and Snack Ideas**................... 23

CHAPTER 6.. 27
MAXIMIZING WORKOUTS.......................... 27
❖ **Effective Exercise Strategies**....................... 27

CHAPTER 7.. **33**
Tracking Progress... **33**
❖ **Keeping a Food Diary and Measuring Success.**
33

CHAPTER 8...**39**
OVERCOMING CHALLENGES........................**39**
❖ **Dealing with Cravings and Staying Motivated..**
39

CHAPTER 9.. **45**
SUCCESS STORIES...**45**
❖ **Real-Life Inspirations**...............................**45**

CHAPTER 10.. **49**
FAQ and TIPS...**49**
❖ **Common Questions and Pro Tips**............... **49**

CONCLUSION...**55**

INTRODUCTION

We're happy you're here at "Carb Cycling for Weight Loss for Women Endomorph: A Guide for Endomorph Women."

Are you an endomorph lady wanting to start a path to greater fitness, health, and long-term weight management? If so, you've chosen the appropriate manual.

Being an endomorph has its own special set of difficulties, but it also has amazing capabilities and possibilities. This book is a complete road map for using those assets and overcoming any challenges that may arise.

You will discover a wealth of knowledge and helpful suggestions geared especially to the requirements of endomorph women in the pages that follow. We'll examine the science of carb cycling and provide a clear grasp of how it might benefit you. You'll learn how to evaluate your current diet, make realistic objectives, choose the correct carbohydrates, create balanced meal plans, and successfully negotiate the world of exercise.

But this manual goes beyond theory. To assist you in overcoming cravings, maintaining motivation, and making long-lasting improvement, we will examine real-life success stories and provide practical advice. It's a wholistic strategy that considers both your physical and psychological well-being.

Carb cycling is not a one-size-fits-all experience for you. This book is your dependable travel companion on your own unique trip. The techniques you'll learn here may be customized to match your particular objectives, whether you're trying to lose weight, gain strength, or just live a better lifestyle.

So let's start this adventure together. You have the ability to change your life and embrace a healthier, happier version of yourself with the proper information, techniques, and steadfast resolve. Let's get started with the effective method of carb cycling to help you succeed as an endomorph lady.

CHAPTER 1

UNDERSTANDING ENDOMORPHS

❖ *What Makes You an Endomorph?*

Being an endomorph means having a unique body type with certain physical characteristics and metabolic tendencies. If you consider yourself to be an endomorph, it's important to comprehend the following:

1. hereditary Predisposition to Store Body Fat Efficiently: Compared to people with other body types, endomorphs have a hereditary tendency to store body fat more effectively. As a consequence, fat may accumulate largely in the hips, thighs, and lower abdomen, giving the body a rounder or softer appearance.

2. Fuller Figure: The body profile of endomorphs is often curvier or more pear-shaped. This entails having larger hips and a smaller waist, which helps one seem voluptuous naturally.

3. Weight Management Challenges: Due to their intrinsic propensity to store fat, endomorphs may find it more difficult to maintain or lose weight. To lose weight and maintain a healthy body composition, one may need to take a more concentrated and systematic approach.

4. Slower Metabolism: Endomorphs often have a metabolism that burns calories more slowly than ectomorphs (body types with slim physiques). It may be simpler to acquire weight and more difficult to lose extra pounds due to this reduced metabolic rate.

5. Strong Lower Body Muscles: Having naturally well-developed leg and glute muscles is a benefit of being an endomorph. This may increase strength and power, especially when working the lower body.

Understanding your endomorph body type is essential to customizing your diet and exercise routine to suit your individual needs and objectives. You may work toward developing a healthy and balanced body while optimizing your talents by accepting your inherent characteristics and putting the right tactics into practice.

CHAPTER 2

THE POWER OF CARB CYCLING

❖ *How Carb Cycling Helps Endomorph Women*

Dietary strategies like carb cycling may be very helpful for endomorph women who want to control their weight and enhance their general health. How carb cycling may benefit endomorph women is as follows:

1. Metabolic Flexibility: By alternating between days with high and low carbohydrate intake, carb cycling promotes metabolic flexibility. Your body is forced to adapt to various fuel sources as a result of this variance, making it more adept at using both carbs and fats as fuel. This flexibility may improve calorie use and fat burning for endomorphs whose metabolisms typically have a slower rate.

2. Regulated Insulin Levels: Endomorphs often have increased insulin sensitivity, which may result in fat accumulation. By limiting carbohydrate consumption on some days, carb cycling controls insulin levels. This makes it simpler for endomorph women to regulate their weight by lowering insulin surges, stabilizing blood sugar, and minimizing fat accumulation.

3. Fat Loss and Muscle Preservation: The body uses more fat reserves for energy on low-carb days, which encourages fat loss. In addition, enough protein consumption throughout these stages aids in maintaining lean muscle mass, which is essential for enhancing metabolism and developing a toned body.

4. Energy Balance: Carb cycling offers a balanced method for consuming energy. Days with a lot of carbohydrates provide the energy needed for demanding exercises and replenishing glycogen reserves, while days with few carbohydrates promote fat burning. This balance promotes both fat reduction objectives and workout performance.

5. Better Hormonal Balance: Hormonal abnormalities might interfere with weight control for many endomorph women. Leptin and ghrelin, two hormones that affect hunger and appetite, may be controlled by carb cycling. The use of carb cycling may lower cravings and overeating by controlling these hormones.

6. Versatile Dietary Strategy: Carb cycling is a versatile and durable dietary strategy. It makes it psychologically simpler to stick to

long-term since it allows for occasional indulgences on days when you eat a lot of carbs. For endomorph women who want to maintain a healthy weight and way of life, this sustainability is essential.

The bottom line is that carb cycling gives endomorph women the ability to adjust their metabolism, insulin sensitivity, and overall body composition. Endomorphs may accomplish their fitness and weight reduction objectives while also enjoying a more well-balanced and manageable nutritional approach by deliberately varying their carbohydrate intake.

CHAPTER 3

STARTING YOUR CARB CYCLING JOURNEY

❖ *Assessing Your Current Diet and Goals*

Endomorph women should assess their existing eating patterns and establish specific, attainable objectives before starting a carb cycling adventure. An effective carb cycling strategy based on individualized requirements and preferences is built on the results of this evaluation step. The first step is as follows:

Keep a comprehensive note of the food you eat every day for at least a week to start. Include the portions and time of each meal, as well as everything you eat and drink. Your eating habits, calorie intake, and the kinds of foods you often eat will all be revealed by this journal.

2. Review Your Eating Patterns: Look back through your food journal to identify any patterns or repeated habits. Pay attention to times when you overeat high-calorie, low-nutrient foods, indulge mindlessly, or eat out of emotion. You must first comprehend your current actions in order to make positive changes.

3. Calculate Your Baseline Caloric Intake: Using online calculators or talking to a nutritionist, you may determine how many calories you need each day depending on your age, weight, height, level of exercise, and objectives. Using this information, you may assess if you are presently taking in more or less calories than your body needs.

4. Establish Clear and Realistic objectives: Establish specific objectives for your carb

cycling adventure. These aims might be ones for muscle gain, weight reduction, or bettering general well-being and energy levels. Make sure your objectives are precise, quantifiable, and deadline-driven.

5. Identify Problem Areas: Determine which components of your present diet may need to be adjusted. This can include cutting down on sweets, consuming more vegetables, or finding healthier snacks to replace high-calorie ones.

6. Take into consideration dietary preferences: Consider your dietary needs and preferences. Whether you're vegetarian, have food allergies, or adhere to a particular nutritional philosophy, be sure your carb cycling strategy fits your tastes and dietary needs.

7. Seek Professional Guidance: If you're unsure how to evaluate your diet or choose the right objectives, you may want to speak with a licensed dietitian or nutritionist. To meet your unique requirements, they may provide individualized advice and design a carb cycling regimen.

In addition to assisting you in understanding where you are starting from, evaluating your current diet and establishing specific objectives will also provide you a roadmap for your path toward carb cycling. As you continue carb cycling for weight reduction and better health, this self-awareness will enable you to make knowledgeable food decisions and monitor your progress successfully.

CHAPTER 4

CRAFTING YOUR CARB CYCLING DIET

❖ *Choosing Carbs Wisely*

Making educated decisions regarding the kinds of carbs you take is essential for achieving the best outcomes while carb cycling as an endomorph woman. Here is a guide on choose carbohydrates sensibly:

1. Stress Complex carbs: Complex carbs should be prioritized above simple ones. Complex carbohydrates are high in fiber and minerals and may be found in foods like whole grains (such as brown rice, quinoa, and oats), legumes (such as lentils, chickpeas), and vegetables (such as sweet potatoes, broccoli). They help balance blood sugar levels and provide enduring energy, avoiding energy dips and cravings.

Include fibrous vegetables like broccoli, spinach, kale, and cauliflower in your diet. These vegetables are loaded with vitamins and minerals, have a low calorie content, and have a lot of fiber. They enhance digestive health and aid with satiety.

3. Select entire Fruits: Rather than fruit drinks or processed snacks, choose entire fruits. Whole fruits include fiber, which reduces the rate at which sugar is absorbed and aids in maintaining stable blood sugar levels. The best options include berries, apples, and citrus fruits.

4. Reduce Refined Carbohydrate Intake: Reduce the amount of refined carbs you consume, such as white bread, sugary cereals, and pastries. For endomorphs in particular, these meals may cause quick

blood sugar rises and increased fat accumulation.

5. Watch Portion Sizes: Watch your portions, particularly on days when you consume a lot of carbohydrates. Even while you need healthy carbs in your diet, eating too much of them might result in an excess of calories that you don't need.

6. Time Your Carbs Strategically: Space out your daily carbohydrate consumption. When your body can utilize them for energy and recuperation, around your exercises is a good time to consume more of your regular carbohydrate intake.

7. Experiment with Different Carb Sources: To keep your diet interesting, try out different carb sources. To avoid becoming

bored and to maintain a varied intake of nutrients, try adding various grains, beans, and veggies.

8. Carefully study food labels before selecting any packaged goods. Look for foods that include a lot of fiber and little added sugars. Choose products that ideally have few, recognized components.

9. Maintain Adequate Hydration: Proper hydration is necessary for effective carbohydrate metabolism. Enough water consumption promotes general health and aids in the efficient digestion of carbohydrates by the body.

10. Listen to Your Body: Take note of how certain carbs affect your body's reactions. If you discover that a certain meal causes

bloating, pain, or energy slumps, think about tailoring your diet to your unique requirements.

Making appropriate carbohydrate choices is a key component of an effective carb cycling diet for endomorph women. You can help stabilize your blood sugar levels, preserve energy, and encourage fat reduction while consuming a balanced and delicious meal by choosing nutrient-dense, fiber-rich alternatives and paying attention to portion sizes.

CHAPTER 5

Meal Plans Made Easy

❖ *Sample Meals and Snack Ideas*

For endomorph women, creating nutritious, delectable meals and snacks is essential to a successful carb cycling regimen. Here are some example carb cycling meal and snack ideas to get you started:

Daytime High-Carb Meals:

1. Breakfast:
- Fresh berries and honey drizzled on top of oatmeal.
- Banana slices with almond butter on whole-grain bread.

2. Lunch:
- Salad of quinoa with chickpeas, mixed veggies, and a lemon-tahini dressing.

- Wraps made of tofu or turkey and whole-grain tortillas are loaded with vibrant vegetables.

3. Dinner:
- Fish baked in the oven with quinoa and vegetables on the side.
- With a side of mixed greens, sweet potato and black bean chili is served.

Daytime Low-Carb Meals:

1. Breakfast:
- Feta cheese, spinach, and scrambled eggs.
- Greek yogurt parfait with some strawberries, walnuts, and chia seeds.

2. Lunch:

- Salad of grilled tofu or chicken with cucumber, mixed greens, and vinaigrette dressing.
- lean ground turkey with zucchini noodles (zoodles) in a tomato-based sauce.

3. Dinner:
- Quinoa and asparagus with baked cod or tempeh as a side dish.
- Tofu stir-fried with bell peppers, broccoli, and a mild soy-ginger sauce.

Ideas for Snacks (both Days):

1. Low-Fat Snacks:

- An apple cut into slices and a spoonful of almond butter.
- Greek yogurt topped with honey and oats.

- A tiny handful of assorted dried fruits and nuts.

2. Healthy Snacks:
- Cherry tomatoes, cottage cheese, and a little black pepper.
- Hummus with cucumber slices.
- uncooked eggs.

Snack Tip: To aid with muscle maintenance and satiety, including protein-rich snacks on both high- and low-carb days.

Don't forget to customize these suggested ideas to fit your dietary restrictions and tastes. Variety, balance, and moderation are the secrets to effective carb cycling. To assist you reach your objectives while taking pleasure in a varied and delicious diet, adjust your meals and snacks to ensure that they correspond with your particular high-carb and low-carb days.

CHAPTER 6

MAXIMIZING WORKOUTS

❖ *Effective Exercise Strategies*

Endomorph women who want to lose weight and get in shape need to complement their carb cycling diet with the appropriate workout techniques. Here are some suggestions for efficient workout methods:

1. Combining cardio and strength training is a good idea.

- Include both strength training (weight lifting, resistance bands, bodyweight exercises) and aerobic workouts (like jogging, cycling, or swimming) in your program. Strength training helps you create lean muscle, which increases your metabolism, while cardio improves cardiovascular health and burns calories.

2. Exercise that involves high-intensity bursts (HIIT):

- Short bursts of intensive activity are interspersed with fast rest intervals during HIIT exercises. These sessions may assist boost your metabolism for hours after your exercise and are highly effective at burning fat.

3. Resistance Exercise to Build Muscle:

- Make resistance exercise a priority to increase and preserve your muscle mass. Lean muscle is advantageous for weight control since it helps to tone the body and burns more calories when at rest.

4. Concentrate on Compound Motions:
- Squats, deadlifts, and bench presses are examples of compound exercises that work many muscular groups at once. These activities enhance calorie expenditure while fostering general muscular growth and strength.

5. Core Stabilization:
- Stability and balance depend on a solid core. To strengthen your stomach, use core workouts like planks, Russian twists, and leg lifts.

6. Flexible Exercise Routine:
- Conveniently time your workouts to go along with your carb cycling days. You

may work out harder on days when you eat more carbohydrates, but low-carb days may be better suited to active recuperation or lower-intensity activities.

7. Recurrence and Advancement:
- Long-term fitness objectives must be met consistently. Keep a record of your exercises, progressively increase the intensity, and set challenging goals for yourself to meet. This may assist keep progress going and avoid plateaus.

8. Rest and Recovery Days:
- Give your body enough time to rest. Days of rest are essential for repairing muscles and avoiding burnout. Pay attention to your body's needs and don't be afraid to rest when necessary.

9. Advice from Professionals:

- If you're new to exercising or want to improve your methods, think about speaking with a fitness coach or trainer. They may assist you in developing a customized exercise schedule that complements your carb cycling plan and goals.

10. Mindfulness Training:

- Pay attention to how you feel after exercising. Make exercise a sustainable and pleasurable part of your lifestyle by engaging in activities you like. This may support your continued motivation and reliability.

Remember that your eating habits and general way of life have a big impact on how successful your workout plan is. Endomorph women may maximize their efforts toward reaching their targeted weight reduction and fitness objectives by combining a well-structured training schedule with carb cycling and a healthy diet.

CHAPTER 7

Tracking Progress

❖ *Keeping a Food Diary and Measuring Success*

A good carb cycling program for endomorph women requires keeping a meal journal and setting up techniques to gauge your progress. Following are some tips for using a food diary to measure your progress:

Keep a Food Journal:

Write down everything you eat and drink during the day. This includes every meal and snack. Include the ingredients, cooking techniques, and portion quantities. Be frank and accurate in your entries.

Observe the Timing: Keep track of the times you eat your meals and snacks. This might make it easier to see any trends in your desires and appetite.

Include Details: Write down the restaurant or brand names, as well as any relevant nutritional information, whether you consume packaged food or go out to a restaurant. This will give you a complete picture of your eating preferences.

Track Your Fluid consumption: Be sure to keep an eye on your fluid consumption. Keep track of how much water, tea, coffee, or other liquids you drink every day.

Keep a record of emotional eating and be mindful of its causes. Keep track of any times you overate as a result of stress, boredom, or other feelings. You may discover trends and create better coping mechanisms thanks to this.

Measurement of Success

Scale and measures: To monitor changes in your weight and body composition over time, weigh yourself often and take body measures (waist, hips, and thighs). Remember that swings are common; thus, pay more attention to patterns than to daily figures.

Progress Pictures: To visually monitor your progress, take "before" pictures when you first begin your carb cycling strategy and fresh pictures from time to time. Changes in your body might sometimes take longer to show up on the scale.

Fitness milestones: Track advancements in your level of fitness. Keep track of your accomplishments, such as gains in strength, longer training sessions, or more endurance. These little successes might inspire you and show that you're making progress.

Mood and Energy Levels: Pay attention to changes in your mood and energy levels. On days when you eat a lot of carbohydrates, you could feel more energized than on days when you eat less. Success may also be indicated by an uptick in mood, attentiveness, and sleep quality.

Hunger & Cravings: Pay attention to how they alter. You could have less cravings for sweet or calorie-dense meals as your body becomes used to carb cycling, as well as better appetite control.

Following your carb cycling strategy consistently is a crucial component of success. Celebrate maintaining your food and exercise schedules since consistency is key to long-term success.

Consult a Professional: If you have particular health objectives or concerns, think about speaking with a qualified nutritionist or fitness professional who can provide professional advice and assist you in correctly tracking your progress.

Keep in mind that there will always be setbacks and that development may not always be linear. As an endomorph lady embarking on a carb cycling journey, you may remain motivated, see areas for development, and make required modifications to reach your intended objectives by keeping a food diary and monitoring performance in several ways.

CHAPTER 8

OVERCOMING CHALLENGES

❖ *Dealing with Cravings and Staying Motivated*

Success in carb cycling for endomorph women depends on controlling cravings and staying motivated. Here are some methods to help you resist urges and stick with your objectives:

How to Manage Cravings:

Identify Triggers: Be aware of what makes you want certain foods. Is it anxiety, boredom, or certain dietary cues? Finding your triggers will help you develop healthy coping mechanisms.

Plan your meals and abide by your carb cycling diet. Blood sugar levels may be stabilized and cravings can be decreased with regular, balanced meals that include a variety of complex carbs, proteins, and healthy fats.

Keep Hydrated: Sometimes, hunger and thirst are confused. To stay well hydrated throughout the day, drink plenty of water.

Include Satisfying items: Include tastier items that satiate your appetites. For instance, choose a piece of dark chocolate or a fruit smoothie with a dash of honey if you're craving sweets.

Eat mindfully by focusing on the tastes and sensations of your meal. You may enjoy your meals more and resist the impulse to overeat by eating attentively.

Maintain a stock of wholesome snacks for easy access. To satisfy appetites in between meals, choose alternatives like carrot sticks with hummus, Greek yogurt with berries, or a handful of mixed nuts.

Portion control: Give yourself a modest serving if you're seeking a less healthful food. The secret to avoiding deprivation is moderation.

Maintaining Motivation

Set Achievable and Realistic objectives: Make sure your objectives are both. Divide them into minor accomplishments to acknowledge along the road.

Visualize Success: Picture the advantages of achieving your objectives. Motivation might be increased by imagining yourself fitter and healthier.

Accountability: Tell a friend or family member your objectives so they can encourage you and hold you responsible.

Track Progress: Keep an eye on your development, whether it is by measurements, pictures, or physical accomplishments. Realistic outcomes may be quite motivating.

Set up a system of prizes for achieving milestones to reward yourself. Spend some time at the spa, get new gym clothing, or go to the movies as incentives instead of eating them.

fitness Variety: Try new exercises or classes to keep your fitness regimen interesting. Boredom may be avoided, and variety can keep people motivated.

Consider joining a community online or for fitness enthusiasts. With those who have similar interests, it may be motivating and supportive to share experiences and progress.

Recall your motivation for beginning your carb cycling adventure when you reflect on it. Reconnect with your motivations on a regular basis, whether it's for better health, more energy, or more confidence.

Recognize that setbacks are a normal part of any journey as you learn from them. Instead of being disheartened, use the opportunity to learn from failures and become stronger.

counsel from a professional: If you're having trouble staying motivated or are uncertain about your strategy, go to a qualified dietitian or personal trainer who can provide you with support and individualized counsel.

You may stick to your carb cycling plan as an endomorph woman by using these methods to deal with cravings and keep your motivation up, eventually reaching your weight reduction and fitness objectives.

CHAPTER 9

SUCCESS STORIES

❖ *Real-Life Inspirations*

A strong incentive for your carb cycling journey as an endomorph lady may be found in real-life success tales. These tales serve as a reminder that with hard work and determination, accomplishing our objectives is not only conceivable but also achievable. Here are a few motivational instances:

1. Transformation Tales: Many endomorph women have shared their transformational tales, displaying their success with carb cycling in terms of fitness and weight reduction. Before-and-after pictures that describe the difficulties encountered and the actions done to overcome them are often included in these tales.

2. Look to successful athletes who are endomorphs in their respective sports. Their devotion to exercise, diet, and self-control may serve as an inspiration for what is possible when one is committed.

3. Role models and celebrities: Some prominent figures and celebrities are endomorphs who follow healthy lives. Their candor regarding their eating and exercise habits may encourage others to do the same.

4. Support from the community: Endomorph women have forums and social media platforms where they may talk about their achievements, difficulties, and victories. Joining these communities may be a terrific way to get inspiration and support.

5. Personal Connections: Friends, family members, or acquaintances who have successfully adopted carb cycling or other fitness techniques sometimes have the most encouraging tales to share. Hearing about their own journeys may be inspiring and relevant.

6. Everyday Heroes: People who have made substantial adjustments to better their health and wellbeing are considered everyday heroes. These examples show that, whatever one's starting place, change is possible for everyone.

7. Health Improvements: Motivational tales don't always revolve on physical beauty or weight loss. Some people talk about their paths to greater health, including how they've managed their medical illnesses, gained more energy, and improved their emotional wellbeing.

8. Overcoming Obstacles: It may be very inspiring to read about how others have overcome difficulties, disappointments, and plateaus. It demonstrates how persistence is often the secret to long-term success.

Always keep in mind that everyone's path is different while looking for inspiration. It's possible that what works for one individual is different for another. Use these true tales as motivation, but adjust your strategy to fit your objectives, preferences, and environment. As you go along your carb cycling journey, you may write your own motivational tale if you are persistent and determined.

CHAPTER 10

FAQ and TIPS

❖ *Common Questions and Pro Tips*

As an endomorph lady, navigating the world of carb cycling may be complicated and difficult. Here are some frequently asked questions and expert advice to assist you:

Typical Questions

1. Are endomorphs safe to cycle carbohydrates?

- Yes, when done properly, carb cycling may be both safe and beneficial for endomorphs. Before beginning any new diet plan, it is important to speak with a healthcare professional or nutritionist, particularly if you have underlying medical issues.

2. How often should I alternate carbs?

- Having high-carb days and low-carb days is a frequent carb cycling strategy, however the frequency might vary. Although some people adhere to a 3:1 or 2:1 ratio of low-carb to high-carb days, it's important to adjust the program to fit your unique requirements and tastes.

3. What should I eat when my carb intake is high?

- Focus on complex carbohydrates like whole grains, lentils, and starchy vegetables when you're eating a lot of carbs. To produce balanced meals, include lean meats and healthy fats.

4. Can I indulge on days when I'm not carb cycling?

- Even if the odd indulgence is allowed, it's important to avoid having too many cheat days since they might hinder your progress. Plan these days carefully and wisely.

5. How can I avoid cravings while eating low carb?

- On low-carb days, make sure you're eating enough protein- and fiber-rich items to keep you full and content. Cravings may also be managed by drinking plenty of water and having healthy fats in your meals.

Pro Advice:

1. Make Your Plan Specific: Adapt your carb cycling strategy to your own objectives, amount of exercise, and preferences. There isn't a method that works for everyone.

2. Track Your Macros: Pay careful attention to the amount of protein, carbs, and fats you consume each day. You may adjust your strategy in light of this to get the best outcomes.

3. Stay Consistent: The secret to carb cycling success is consistency. Maintain your routine despite difficulties or hectic days.

4. Plan and Prepare: Make your meals and snacks in advance, particularly on days when you are eating low-carb.

Having convenient access to wholesome alternatives may help people avoid making hasty, unhealthy decisions.

5. Take Note of Your Body: Observe how your body reacts to carb cycling. If you feel excessive exhaustion, cravings, or other negative consequences, change your strategy.

6. Combine Carb Cycling with Exercise: To optimize the advantages of carb cycling, include regular exercise into your daily regimen. Exercises that combine cardio and strength training may be very beneficial.

7. Continue learning about nutrition and carb cycling to stay informed. A

crucial tool for making wise decisions is knowledge.

8. Seek Support: Discuss your trip with a friend, member of your family, or a community online. Having a support network may help with accountability and motivation.

Keep in mind that carb cycling is a flexible strategy, and it could take some trial and error to determine what works best for you. As an endomorph lady embarking on a carb cycling adventure, be patient, be dedicated to your objectives, and don't be afraid to change your diet when necessary to get the outcomes you want.

CONCLUSION

It's crucial to remain focused and keep moving forward as an endomorph lady as you continue your carb cycling adventure. What comes next and how to keep moving forward are as follows:

1. Make your carb cycling plan more precise:

Continually evaluate and improve your carb cycling plan. To better meet your objectives, you may need to modify the frequency of high- and low-carb days, adjust your macronutrient ratios, or adjust your meal planning.

2. Set fresh targets:

It's time to create new objectives once you've accomplished your previous ones. These can concern accelerating weight reduction, gaining muscle, enhancing exercise performance, or improving general health and wellbeing.

3. Put an effort forth:

Continue to push yourself throughout your exercises. To remain motivated and keep improving, gradually raise the intensity, try out new exercises, or create personal fitness goals.

4. Watch and Adjust:

Keep a regular record of your weight, measurements, and physical accomplishments to track your progress. Make educated changes to your carb cycling and workout regimens using this data.

5. Accept Variety:

Keep your diet and workout regimen varied. To avoid boredom and plateaus, try new meals, recipes, and exercise techniques.

6. Emphasis on sustainability and good health

Change your attention from immediate outcomes to long-term sustainability and wellness. Carb cycling ought to be a way of life rather than a passing fad. Aim for a healthy, nutrient-rich diet that is well-balanced.

7. Pay Attention to Your Body:

Pay attention to the cues from your body. Consider changing your plan if you feel extreme exhaustion, constant cravings, or other negative consequences.

8. Highlight Successes:

Celebrate your accomplishments as you go. Recognize and reward your efforts if you achieve a weight milestone, achieve a personal best during a workout, or consistently follow your plan.

9. Seek Advice from a Professional:

Do not be afraid to speak with a licensed nutritionist, personal trainer, or healthcare professional if you are having difficulties or have particular health and fitness concerns. They are able to provide tailored help and recommendations.

10. Remain Inspired:

Keep in touch with the things that motivate you, whether they were your starting points or your accomplishments. Find a group of friends or online forums that are supportive and strive for the same things.

Keep in mind that the process of carb cycling is dynamic. Accept lifelong learning, be flexible, and stay dedicated to reaching your fitness and health objectives. You may use carb cycling as a strategy for success if you remain committed and proactive throughout your journey as an endomorph lady.

www.ingramcontent.com/pod-product-compliance
Lightning Source LLC
Chambersburg PA
CBHW061933270726
48660CB00007BA/2706